DENISE BENNER

I0437026

YOU ARE
Not Alone

(EVEN IF YOU THINK YOU ARE)

*A little book of stories, support, and advice
through the journey of dementia care*

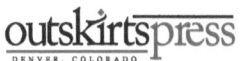

DENVER, COLORADO

You Are Not Alone (Even if You Think You Are)
A little book of stories, support, and advice through the journey of dementia care
All Rights Reserved.
Copyright © 2015 Denise Benner
v4.0

Outskirts Press, Inc.
http://www.outskirtspress.com

ISBN: 978-1-4787-4917-2

Outskirts Press and the "OP" logo are trademarks belonging to Outskirts Press, Inc.

PRINTED IN THE UNITED STATES OF AMERICA

"KINDRED SPIRITS ARE NOT SO SCARCE AS I USED TO THINK.
IT'S SPLENDID TO FIND OUT THERE ARE SO MANY OF
THEM IN THE WORLD"
-L.M. Montgomery, Anne of Green Gables

I dedicate this book to my parents.

*They taught me the importance of love,
devotion, and happiness.*

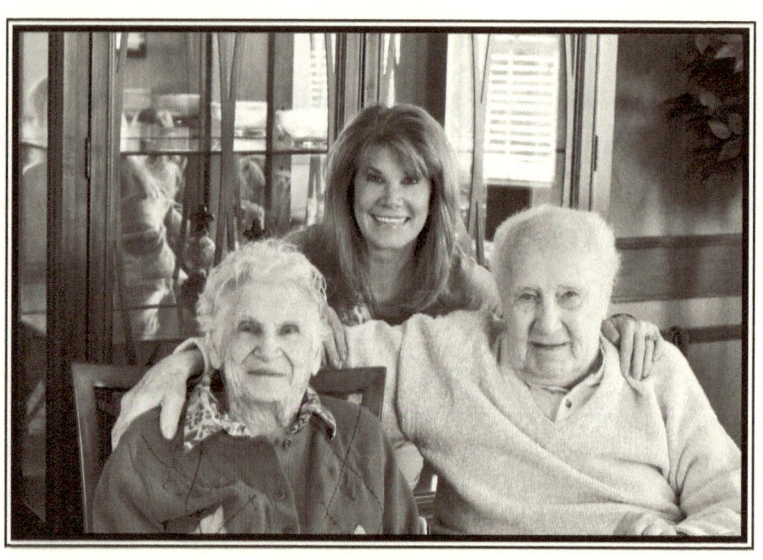

30 Years Later

Years ago, I bought diapers for my child.

30 years later, I'm buying diapers for my parents.

Years ago, I pushed my child in a stroller.

30 years later, I'm pushing my parent in a wheelchair.

Years ago, I didn't leave home without the stroller in the trunk of my car.

30 years later, I don't leave home without a wheelchair in the trunk of my car.

Years ago, it was a battle to get my child to shower.

30 years later, it is a battle to get my parent to shower.

Years ago, my child would say, "Can't 'member, Mom!"

30 years later, my parent says, "I can't remember."

Denise Benner 2014

PREFACE

My parents met in 1939, when she was 16 and he, 18. Both will tell you the story, with my dad singing, "Standing on the corner, watching all the girls go by..." He frequently watched my mom go by the corner where he and his buddies would stand. One day, he said to her, "I've got a dime, and if you have the balance, we can go to the drugstore and get a soda." My mom later said, "It was that first date, we knew we would be together."

Fast forward to the fall of 2005. My dad, at age 85, was diagnosed with Alzheimer's Disease. The doctor only did a few tests with my dad, before she pronounced the diagnosis, which I found surprising. "Mr. Paul, you have Alzheimer's." The cold in those words made the chill in the air palpable. The expression on my dad's face was one I will never forget. His look was devastation and shock.

I couldn't accept the diagnosis. Maybe I was in denial. I spoke with a friend of mine, who is a physician. She arranged for my dad to see a memory specialist in Columbia, South Carolina, where I live. The specialist sat with my dad for 2 1/2 hours. He put my dad through an array of tests and talked at length with my dad. His conclusion was my dad did not have Alzheimer's Disease but, at age 85, had symptoms of dementia.

Even though the specialist kept encouraging my dad

to keep performing his daily routine, my dad practically gave up living his life. He never forgot the icy words: "You have Alzheimer's." He is a very intelligent man who always had control of his destiny. He no longer had that control. He was embarrassed when he would forget people's names. He would forget why he was supposed to be somewhere. Sadly, he shut himself inside his own home and within himself.

My mom tried to bring my dad to her social functions. She felt she could help him if he became confused. He agreed. However, that was short lived. He felt very awkward, and his comfort level was to be in his home.

As time passed, my mom stopped going to her social events. I found out from one of her friends that she was getting lost driving to different functions. Instead of admitting her confusion, she simply stopped going out. My mom would make up "excuses" for not going to her activities. She was always very socially active. This was not normal for her.

I called her doctor and asked for him to see her. At the same age my dad was developing symptoms of dementia, my mom was also. Both, at age 85, had the symptoms of dementia.

It has been quite the journey.

I have always been very close to my parents. They were always there for me. Now, it is my turn to be there for them. My dad has been my hero, and it has been very difficult watching both of them decline in memory, thinking and reasoning skills. Nonetheless, the joy I see in the love they share is priceless. They can't remember what they had for breakfast, lunch or dinner. However, they still remember what it is to love.

Throughout this journey with my parents, I have encountered people who are also confronted with the reality of loved ones who have some form of dementia. Many people will open up and start comparing stories. It is as though we have our own community, a kindred spirit.

Listening to their stories made me realize that our experiences and stories needed to be shared. So many of us feel we are struggling, at times, alone. But we really aren't alone.

I hope you will relate and find comfort in reading the heartfelt personal stories and advice from caregivers I have had the pleasure to meet.

Denise Benner
November, 2014

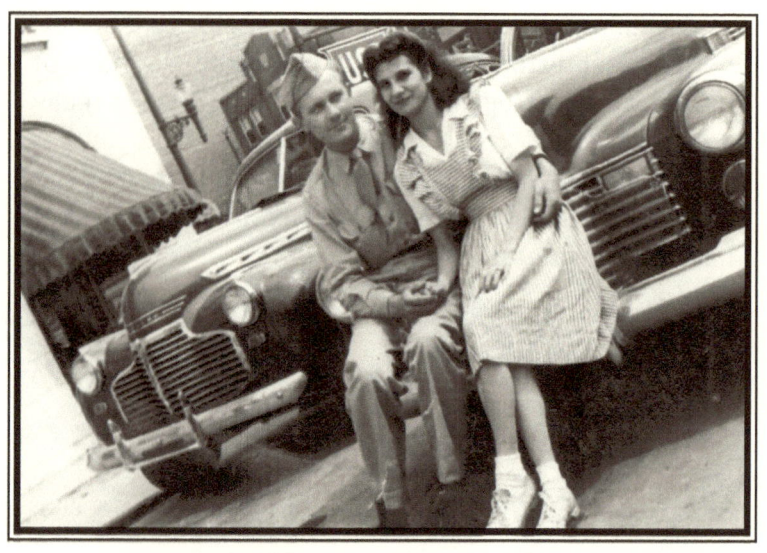

Wedding Day: July 3, 1943

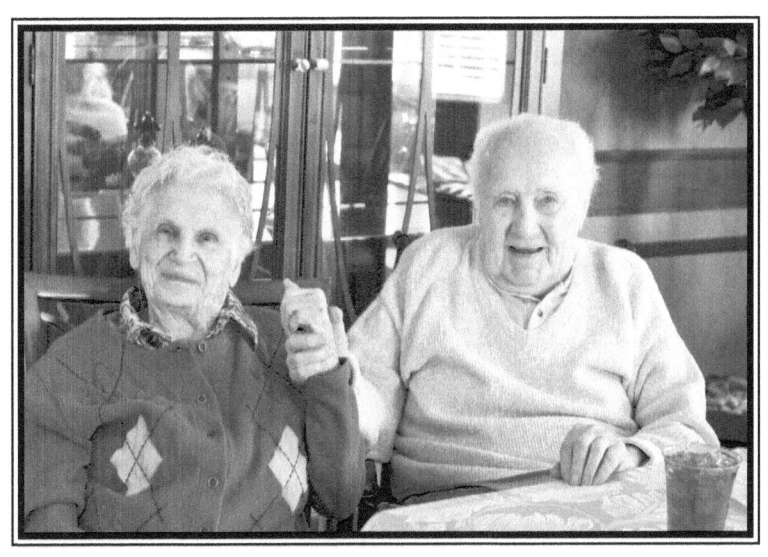

July 3, 2014

ACKNOWLEDGMENTS:

I want to thank all those who took the time to share their stories. I formed bonds that will remain in my heart for a lifetime.

To Kristen, Jesse, Eleanor, Meredith, Adam and Lauren, I thank you for your love and support.

A very special thank you to my loving husband, Chris, for his patience, comfort and heart.

TABLE OF CONTENTS

Chapter
One

DENIAL

Denial can come from the person who has dementia and from family members, as well.

Many people are very good at hiding their symptoms of dementia.

Be patient with person who is in denial. It is a part of a grieving process many of us will go through.

For those suffering with and those with a loved one with dementia or Alzheimer's Disease, it is very difficult to process what lies ahead for them.

"How could this happen? It can't be true!" Acceptance is burdensome for all those involved.

As caregivers, we know it won't get better. As dementia progresses, let the person know you love them. And know that they will never stop loving you.

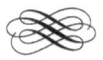

MARGARET'S STORY:

My first hint that there were issues with my mother's memory was during a discussion about trips she wished she had been able to take. I reminded her that my sister and I had taken her to New York City a few months prior. She had no memory of it.

My mother would get lost driving to her doctors' appointments. She would have to return home to find the address in the her phone directory to jog her memory. She had always documented her daily blood pressure and blood sugar in her notebook. Yet, when I visited her, I saw she had stopped her daily recordings. She insisted she wrote them down. But, they weren't there.

Around Christmas one year, my mother had a fall. She insisted it was nothing. I lived a couple of hours from her, and her neighbor drove her to our home to stay with us for the holidays. I was shocked when I saw the bruising on her face. She looked like she had been beaten. That was the final indication that she could no longer live alone.

After the holidays, we visited retirement homes close by. My mother agreed to move closer to me, and we selected one together. However, days later, she didn't remember any of that. She couldn't believe we were going to move her from her home. She was independent and wanted to remain independent. There was nothing wrong with her, she insisted!

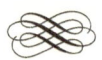

BRENDA' STORY:

My mom is 84 years old. She was married for 35 years, with three children.

She earned a degree in accounting, and in her later years, she decided to return to school and earn her law degree. She was a practicing attorney until she was 79 years old.

Ever since I left home for college, I called my mom at least once a week. For years, I didn't notice anything was wrong with her memory. She, of course, didn't think anything was wrong. Or, she just kept it well hidden.

When visiting her, we had gone out to a local restaurant. When we were through eating, I noticed my mom taking one of the spoons from the table and putting it in her purse. When I asked her about it, she told me not to worry; she was going to return the spoon. This made absolutely no sense. I didn't want to draw attention to us, so I said nothing. This should have been the first "red flag."

During that visit, I noticed my once very social mom had become very isolated. Her seclusion worried me. Because we lived a long distance from my mom, my husband and I suggested she consider moving to our home. My husband wrote her an endearing letter, letting her know she had an open invitation. She refused. She didn't feel the need.

Several weeks after returning home, I received a call that my mom had been in a serious car accident. I immediately flew out to be with her. I stayed for a month, and it was during that period of time that I really began noticing "out of the norm" behavior from her. At first, I attributed it to the accident. I kept wondering whether she would be back to her normal self once she recovered.

When her doctors cleared her to travel, I finally convinced her to move to my home. I needed to return to my family, and I couldn't leave her by herself. One minute she would be "all there"; the next her thoughts would divert completely. It was clear how the accident happened. After finally telling my mom it would be a temporary stay, I gained her consent to return with me.

DANIEL'S STORY:

My mother was in complete denial, but my father was showing the signs and symptoms of dementia. He was forgetful. He would get lost driving. He was becoming depressed. He began to isolate himself. However, she did not want to accept where these signs were pointing.

At that time, they had been married for 65 years. How could the self-made man she had been married to for so long, suddenly change so much? She could not understand his mental decline. I don't think she really wanted to, because that would have meant she had to accept that something was wrong with her husband.

During one of my visits, my mother finally admitted to me how afraid she was of the unknown and of getting old. I realized then that her denial was because of her fear.

I have known family members who will make excuses for their loved ones in cognitive and behavioral decline. They will insist that it was just a bad day, and that everyone has bad days. I now know, the reality is very hard to face.

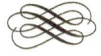

Chapter
Two

ANGER

You, as the caregiver, may have to deal with anger from both ends. Anger within yourself and anger from the person who has dementia.

The anger within ourselves is the emotion we feel towards what has happened, what is happening. You may be angry for the mere fact this decline is happening to the person you love. You may get angry because what you are doing for the person just doesn't seem to be enough. This is normal.

It is also normal for the person with dementia to lash out at you. Remember they may also be angry. The emotional roller coaster within their mind is out of their control. Their fate is no longer theirs to control.

It's hard, I know. Calling your Alzheimer's Association chapter can put you in touch with support groups in your area. Their Website is: www.alz.org, and their toll-free 24/7 helpline is: 800-272-3900.

If there isn't a support group in your area, a good friend who will allow you to vent is priceless!

Journaling is also good for your emotional health. Writing about why you are angry can help you detox the inner struggle that is causing your anger.

When the person with dementia becomes angry, ask yourself what is causing the anger. Sometimes it is beyond your control. Sometimes you can learn how to make the journey less frustrating for him or her. You may have to be creative and think outside of the box to deter an angry outcome.

CYNTHIA'S STORY:

She would lash out. At first, I would argue with her and try to correct her. Afterwards, I would just feel guilty. Shortly thereafter I would be glad, when she would soon forget.

Now, if she is angry, I turn it all into a game, act silly, and get her to laugh. The issue is soon forgotten. This is sometimes easier said than done. I am not always in the "mood" to play games and laugh. This entire situation saddens me and I realize it is not going to get any better.

I get angry as well. I've decided not to focus on this because, ultimately, it affects me more than it affects anyone else. It's like poison. Once it gets into your system, it spreads quickly.

KARL' STORY:

Upon my arrival of visiting my dad at the assisted living facility, there was not a hello. This is what was said:

"When are you taking me home?
I thought you were coming at 3:00 to take me home.
I need to get out of here. This is no place to live!
I want the comfort of my home!"

What do I say? Do I quickly change the subject? Do I tell him he's not going home? That would be useless. It would only hurt him for that present moment, until he asked again. I knew he wasn't happy with me. I also knew his anger would pass. I needed to be patient. I needed to take a deep breath and breathe!

At the advice of a geriatric nurse, I now ask questions about what he misses about his home. Ironically, when I ask him, he can't remember what he misses. But, he still wants to go home.

Unfortunately, this topic comes up frequently. When he does bring it up, I will sometimes start reminiscing about my childhood with him. Once we start exchanging stories, the conversation will lead to other topics. His insistence of going home will pass.

I take every visit one visit at a time. Sometimes, I leave overwhelmed and a bit broken hearted. Other times, I leave with a spring in my step, just knowing he had a happy day.

KATHLEEN'S STORY:

My mom has always had a difficult time getting rid of things. But now she has taken it to another level!

She hoards newspapers, books from the library, magazines, puzzle books, puzzles, and bananas. Yes, bananas!

I have to go to her room when she is distracted with something, getting dressed, for example. I'll load a large shopping bag with her stashes and run to put back the various items she has taken from the common areas where she lives.

Rather than throw out the overly ripened bananas, I have made more banana bread than you might imagine!

It's a struggle to remove the items she hoards. She's forever in her room. It doesn't take her a long time to get herself dressed, so tactics have to be very fast.

This is where the anger against me enters. When she catches me cleaning or removing items, she scolds me. My mom was always a rule follower. Her sense of fairness is gone.

So is her sense of the rules. Residents are allowed only three library books at a time. She doesn't care if anyone else in the building is able to have a magazine or puzzle book. She will keep forty library books, fifty magazines, six jigsaw puzzles, fifteen puzzles books and six or seven bananas (in various stages of ripeness) in her room at one time.

Her anger and her resentment of rules have been a total change from who she once was.

Chapter

Three

WHERE IS HOME?

No one ever wants to move away from what is comfortable to them. Our home is that comfortable place, where memories have been made. To leave it behind must be very frightening. One is headed to the "unknown" whether it be voluntarily or not.

We, as caregivers, need to find the right balance for ourselves and for the person with dementia.

The best formula, according to the person with dementia is, most likely, staying home. If caregivers can accommodate this, that is wonderful! However, that is not always the case.

If you find yourself in this predicament, there are outreach sources available in your community. Ask your doctor for help. The librarian at your local library can also show you resources. Finally, the Alzheimer's Association, www.alz.org, has a wealth of information to help lead you in the right direction. Their 24/7 helpline is 800-272-3900.

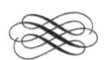

DENISE'S STORY:

My parents retired from Ohio to a beautiful golfing area in North Carolina in 1979. They began to live their dream together.

When my father realized there were health issues on the rise with he and my mother, he wanted to move back to Ohio to be closer to family. My mother refused. All her friends were where they were living, and her social life wouldn't be the same. They stayed in North Carolina. It was important to him for his wife to be happy.

As time passed and my father's memory started to decline, my mother was becoming overwhelmed. Not overwhelmed enough, to move back to Ohio. We all agreed that a part-time caregiver would help alleviate some of her burden. Because of personality conflicts, we had a turnover of several caregivers.

Fortunately, we were finally blessed to find two wonderful women to help with my parents. They stayed with my parents daily for three years. Within those three years, my mother was also diagnosed with dementia.

Health care became an issue. Both had frequent hospital stays. My two siblings discussed moving my parents into assisted living. When both parents heard of this, it was war. After much discussion and debate, we all came to an agreement. My parents would stay in their home with the 24/7 care provided by the two caregivers who were already in place.

That plan lasted two years before I received a phone call that my father broke his hip. He would require surgery as soon as possible.

He came through the surgery with flying colors. However, he was not doing well in rehab. He refused physical therapy. He looked like a dead man lying in his bed. The rehabilitation center wanted to discharge him to a nursing home for skilled and long term care. I was not going to let him vegetate or be moved to skilled care. I knew he had it in him to improve. I wasn't going to leave him alone in a nursing home.

I had moved to South Carolina by that time. I found a rehabilitation center with an assisted living facility next door, which would provide my mother assistance with her daily needs. Within one day, I packed my parents' belongings, scheduled an ambulance transport and with the help of my husband, moved my parents to South Carolina.

In three months, my dad was getting around with a walker or using a wheelchair. He joined my mother in the assisted living facility. Two years in, however, they still think this is a temporary situation.

There are days I visit when they want to know when I'm taking them home. There are days when they insist they go home.

There is no reasoning with either one of them now. I am not sure what to expect with each visit. Will they be happy? Will they want to go home? It's a mystery when I open the door to their little apartment.

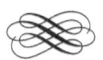

LAURA'S STORY:

Instead of moving my mother-in-law from her home to assisted living, my husband and his siblings decided she would move in with us. I was a former caregiver. Therefore, it made sense for me to take on the responsibility of becoming her primary caregiver.

When the decision was made for my mother-in-law to move to our home, I realized the situation was ideal for me, as it related to "my job." I would be working from home. I could go to another room, go outside, or put in my earbuds, if I needed to take a breather from her continual demands for my attention.

I have come to realize my biggest stress is when my husband, Tom, is home. I can tell he is upset. He will say he feels trapped. He's lost his patience with his mother more than once. When he does, I become frustrated and flustered, knowing he's upset. I cannot manage both of them. When push comes to shove I, literally, shove him out of the room! I have to play referee.

Many days, I deal with my mother-in-law all day, without a break. At first I thought I would get that break when Tom would come home from work. It's reminded me of when I was a new mother. I would count the minutes until my husband arrived home from work so I could relax. Only, now, I don't get that luxury.

I know what I should expect and request from my husband. However, I see his hands shaking when he is buttoning his shirt in the morning. He is very distant most days. How can I demand things from him when I see how this has been affecting him already?

Most of the time, my mother-in-law is extremely easy and compliant. It's the repetition of questions that gnaw at me. She doesn't know if Tom and I know how to handle things correctly. She's always been in control of taking care of herself and everyone else. She still believes she can live in her own home, alone. Because of her dementia, she has lost the ability to reason. It can be exasperating.

This experience has changed me in ways that are different from my experience with my own aging parents, who passed away a few years ago. For example, as much as we take family for granted and we behave at our worst, we know our family will eventually forgive us. I don't have that because she is my mother-in-law. She is not my mother.

This living arrangement has to be a win-win situation. I have to grow in character, modify my behavior, and give up judgement. I just need to do what needs to be done; and move on to my next task in the caring for her, my husband, and, hopefully, myself.

It has become easier for me to put myself into "her" world. I try to encourage my husband to do the same. He is an analytical person and has difficulty with that process. She's his mother on the outside and a child within herself.

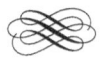

SUZANNE'S STORY:

Life began to change for my husband and I in 1998. My husband, Tony, had bypass surgery. There were some complications after the surgery, which required him to have another surgery. After the second surgery, he had some post-op confusion for a short time. This was the beginning of some personality and behavioral change, but it was very gradual.

Tony's blood pressure started to soar above 200. When this would happen, he would occasionally pass out and then be ok.

We maintained our daily routines for a couple of years. I started to notice he was driving too fast. He would close his eyes while driving. He became sedentary, got angry easily and couldn't complete simple tasks like packing his suitcase. He refused the thought that something might be wrong with him. I insisted we see a neurologist. After an MRI, the neurologist told us there were several white spots in his brain, small strokes.

April 2009 Tony passed out again. After this episode he was very confused and sleepy. I drove him to the emergency room and he was admitted into the hospital. The next day, while visiting him in his hospital room, I witnessed him having a stroke. After this he was unable to walk by himself and had symptoms of Parkinson's Disease. He was diagnosed with multi infarct dementia, which is caused by a series of small strokes.

I had to admit him into a rehab facility. Leaving him there was the worst night of my life. He was confused, scared and angry. He tried to get out the doors and escape. As days passed, he would often sob and want to go home. Sometimes, he thought home was his childhood home and ask about his parents.

After four years of skilled and rehabilitative care, I brought Tony home.

I converted my dining room into his room with a bed, electro lift chair and a wheel chair with card table for eating. I had to secure several doors and the stairs. Tony needs 24/7 attention.

I sleep upstairs with a baby monitor and I have an alarm pad that alerts me if Tony gets up. Fortunately, I have respite care come in the morning for a few hours and in the evening for another few hours.

He is content and interactive most of the time. He is very emotional and cries easily when watching anything sad on the television.

We celebrated our 54th wedding anniversary this year. Each day is a new day with my husband. One day he can be sobbing; and when asked what is wrong, he will tell me he used to know things and now he doesn't. The next day he can be in the bathroom after watching a golf tournament and will be asking, "Where's my ball? It should be here on the green!"

EILEEN'S STORY:

My husband, Frank, graduated with an engineering degree from a prestigious Ivy League college. He attended continuing education classes, even after his retirement, but I started to notice changes in 2006. He stopped attending classes and admitted he wasn't able to keep up with everyone. He had always done our taxes, and in 2007, the IRS sent back our return because of errors.

The decline continued, though. It was slight. He was able to follow the presidential elections, the troubles in the Middle East and crossword puzzles in The New York Times.

Frank broke his hip in 2010. He required three surgeries. With each surgery, I believe the anesthesia and overload of medications slowly made the Frank I knew go away.

His continued decline prompted my children and I to make the decision that Frank needed skilled care I could not provide. We moved him into a long term care facility.

I visit him daily. He is happy. So, I find comfort in that. However, in all honesty, I do miss the Frank I married.

Chapter

Four

CONFLICT

Family conflicts are normal. Unfortunately, family involvement in the care of a person with dementia can cause greater conflict than ever imagined. Different viewpoints on care, childhood issues, control issues and financial matters, for example, can lead to clashes within the family.

Respect and compromise towards the primary caregiver is essential.

Open lines of communication and willingness to compromise can help resolve the conflict amongst family members.

I encourage all those who have a loved one with dementia to attend an Alzheimer's support group. For those who are not the primary caregiver, these support groups can give an insight into the dealings and exasperations the primary caregiver has to face.

Second Wind Dreams® (http://www.secondwind.org/virtual-dementia-tour) offers The Virtual Dementia Tour® as a hands-on experience to help anyone understand the challenges those with dementia face. I recommend all family members to partake in this experience.

MARGARET'S STORY:

One of the saddest parts of my mother's dementia is the relationship she has with my sister. They have never had a good relationship. My sister seems to grow more bitter as time passes. This has become a lose-lose situation for me.

When my sister is with my mother and me, she is rude, dismissive, reprimanding to my mother and cold. She cannot tolerate the mannerisms my mother has developed. Because of this, she doesn't look at our mother. She will argue, she will correct, and she will roll her eyes. It makes for a very uncomfortable situation. She has admitted to me, she "loves" our mother, but she "doesn't like" our mother.

My sister took our mother to my sister's home for Christmas two years ago. It was a disaster for all those in attendance. Because of that, I will never let our mother go to my sister's home for the holidays again, unless I am there.

About every three weeks, my sister drives an hour from her home to take Mother to lunch and shopping. She prefers I go with them, and sometimes I do join them. But, I don't "get a break"! Having her visit, is to allow me a little time on my own. That isn't happening for me.

I do appreciate the money she contributes to help provide for our mother, yet with the tension she brings into the equation, I wonder if it's worth it.

Other people in our family have noticed her sarcasm and angry looks. They can't believe she behaves this way around a person with dementia, but I have been caught in the middle of this for years. I know our mother has no control over some of her behaviors.

My children insisted I move my mother closer to our home, which I did. However, with their busy lives, they don't give me the help I need. I wonder if they also don't know how to deal with her having dementia.

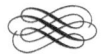

BRENDA'S STORY:

My siblings have decided not to be involved in my mother's care. They have alienated me, and I am not sure if my mother even realizes the abandonment of her two other children. She used to take pride in how well her children got along. They don't write, call or visit, since according to my sister, "It doesn't matter, anyway".

I am very grateful for a supportive husband and children. It is not his responsibility to care for my mother. He has been there for me; he has taken time off of work to help with her; he has done more than any of her other family members, including her two other children.

My siblings have abandoned me in a situation that is out of everyone's control. I believe it's best if my mother doesn't realize this abandonment has happened.

JANIE'S STORY:

I don't sleep anymore. I am in constant worry about my mother and father. I know they are taken care of at the assisted living. However, it bothers me that I am their only visitor. I have wonderful friends who will come with me about once a month or every other month. They all have lost their parents and know what a struggle in can be juggling one's personal life with elderly parents.

I have three siblings who offer little help. They treat my parents' issues as though it were a business. It's all about finances.

Holidays: are what I schedule around my family to make sure my parents have a time with family. That's very important to me, and it puzzles me that it's not important for my siblings.

I have tried to detach myself from my siblings. I don't let them know all I am doing. If I have asked for help from them, they are always too busy. Or, they handle the situation with the attitude of inconvenience. Therefore, I just go and do what's necessary to take care of my parents. It's just not worth it to me to ask for help anymore.

At times, it's very hard visiting my mother and father. I just can't have a pleasant visit with them; each time I'm there, I'm looking for my father's hearing aid, glasses or remote for the television, picking up trash they leave on the floor, hanging clothes in their closet. In general, it's not just a fun visit. The subject always comes up about when they are going home. They don't know where "home" is anymore, but they do know where they are living now is not their home. It breaks my heart.

I try not to worry about them not being showered recently or my dad not being shaved. It's them I am going to see. My mother enjoys the visit. My father will visit for about ten minutes and go back to watching television or sleeping.

I feel very guilty saying what I just did. My mother and father did not ask for any of this. I just wish I had support from the other three children.

NANCY'S STORY:

I am often embarrassed to share my family conflicts with others because I know if my dad were in his right mind, the conflict would not exist. Whenever conflict arose, he would discuss the matter and all would be resolved peacefully.

When my mother passed away, my dad was diagnosed with dementia. He counted on me to do what he wanted. He and I were always two peas in a pod.

Now, that his memory has rapidly declined, I am devastated by the dishonesty of my family members. Financial decisions have been made behind my back. My name was taken off my dad's bank account, unbeknownst to me. Because of this, money was being withdrawn for their vacations and other luxuries! They felt privileged to his bank account because they became primary caregivers to my dad since I moved out of town.

In my heart, I know the financial issues are wrong. What if my dad needs the money for more care in the years to come? Still, I am torn. Would my dad get the attention he deserves from them if the money were not available to them? Would they resent being the primary caregivers? Would they neglect him?

It is such a sad situation.

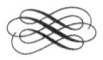

MELANIE'S STORY:

Serenity Prayer
Reinhold Niebuhr (1892-1971)

God grant me the serenity

to accept the things I cannot change;

courage to change the things I can;

and wisdom to know the difference.

Amen.

Don't let anyone who is on the outside, looking in tell you they know how you feel. They don't. They don't bear the burden of the ongoing issues for people with dementia. For example, the doctors' appointments, hospital stays, late night phone calls, phone calls when you go out of town, rearranging your schedule to accommodate for caregiving, or lying awake at night worrying if you are doing everything you can to make your loved ones' lives happy. It can be overwhelming and a weighty burden.

My dear cousin told me to keep reciting the above prayer when in need. Oh, I have repeated this prayer many times!

Because of proximity, I am the family member who takes on the majority of caregiving tasks. Many people think I am an only child, when seen with my parents!

To help save my sanity, I do not have any expectations from my family members. I used to get angry, but I finally came to the conclusion that they don't "get it."

They think they do, and because of that thought process, they will not change. They will always continue not to "get it."

I find it very important to develop relationships with those helping care for our elderly parents. Unfortunately, too many times these important people are undervalued, talked down to, and not respected as they should be. It takes a special and compassionate person to care for the elderly.

I have always had the philosophy in life that things happen for a reason. The responsibilities, sometimes as overwhelming as they can be for me, are mine to have, and this is for a reason.

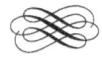

Chapter

Five

GRIEVING

Grief is our emotional response to the loss we feel when the person with dementia is no longer the same person we used to know.

We should allow ourselves to go through the different stages of grieving to reach a point where we can accept our loss and move forward.

www.grief.com outlines the stages of grieving. I quote here a bit from their site in regards to the stages. If you have online access, please go to their Website and read in detail:

DENIAL: "This first stage of grieving helps us to survive the loss".

ANGER: "Anger is a necessary stage of the healing process. Be willing to feel your anger, even though it may seem endless. The more you truly feel it, the more it will begin to dissipate and the more you will heal".

BARGAINING: "Before a loss, it seems like you will do anything if only your loved one would be spared".

DEPRESSION: "After bargaining, our attention moves squarely into the present. Empty feelings present themselves, and grief enters our lives on a deeper level, deeper than we ever imagined".

ACCEPTANCE: "Acceptance is often confused with the notion of being "all right" or "OK" with what has happened. This is not the case. Most people don't ever feel OK or all right about the loss of a loved one. This stage is about accepting the reality."

David Kessler, "The Five Stages of Grief The Responses to Loss That Many People Have". http//www.grief.com/the five-stages/

VICKIE'S STORY:

My dad was my "go-to-man." We always had serious talks. He always had insight and wisdom to share with me. I long for those days. However, I know they are only memories. I have those memories and no one can take them from me.

Presently my dad lives in another state with my other sibling. I would love for him to live with my husband and me, but we move every few years. The change would be a disservice to him and would only confuse his mind more than it is now. I visit him as often as I can.

Despite the fact that, I don't have the dad with whom I shared long conversations, I still have him physically to smother with love and affection when I see him.

I also call him daily. On days I sit on my back porch with my cup of coffee, I describe every detail to him that I can see outside. He loved the outdoors. I describe the trees, the birds chirping, my garden, and whatever else my eyes give glance. I tell him I am having a cup of coffee and imagining he is sitting next to me on the back porch. I believe it gives great comfort to him to listen to my descriptions. I know it brings comfort to me.

I miss my dad. I would love to have my "old dad" back.

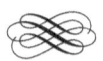

SALLY' STORY:

It's very hard to watch those who had the answers to almost everything no longer have those answers.

I have often wondered which is worse: To lose your loved one in death, while he or she is of right mind, or to watch the decline of the personal being he or she once was.

My son-in-law's 85 year old grandfather passed away in his sleep. When my son-in-law was there to help remove his grandfather's belongings from his retirement condominium, many elderly residents told him how lucky he was to lose his grandfather the way he did. He thought it was a very strange thing to say. I explained to him how lucky he really was. I told him, at that time, I grieved for my dad, even though he was alive. I still have him here, physically, but not mentally.

He is not the same Dad. I lost "my dad" years ago. I miss him. I long for our talks, his laughter, his passion for life.

ALLAN'S STORY:

The roles have been reversed. I often wonder where my mother went. I see her. But, I miss her, because most of the time her mind is not there. I cherish those infrequent lucid moments.

I continue to talk with her, and I share my life experiences and ask for her opinion. I have always loved to make her laugh. I still make that happen!

Recently, she thought I was her brother. But that can't diminish her love. "I really like you. I love you and I can feel that here," she said pointing to her heart.

I know I will miss her dearly the day she leaves this earth. That thought makes me choke up.

This emotional roller coaster is intense at times. It is a long goodbye.

LESLIE'S STORY:

I grieve over the loss of my time and my life. Does that sound selfish? I am 68 years old and have never felt the stress and overwhelming feeling that takes over me. I want my "old life" back!

If my mother were the only recipient of my care taking, I could manage it well. Since she was diagnosed with dementia, I have found most of my time is taking care of her needs. I don't get the time I used to share with my grandchildren. I miss them so much and long for those days when we made cookies, painted, played school and dressed up. They are the light of my life.

My husband is still working full time. He will be retiring soon, and he and I are at the age where we have travel opportunities. I question whether we should continue to take trips, especially out of the country. What if something were to happen to my mother, while we are a long distance away?

We are building a new home, I have friends and an aunt who are ill and I have a mother who needs me. I am overwhelmed with all that is on my plate.

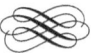

Chapter
Six

MOMENTS

When you are with your loved one, hold hands, smile, sing, play music, look at photos of times past.

Sometimes, these simple acts seem to unlock something in the brain. It can give a glimmer of light. It can bring joy and laughter.

If you try any of the above mentioned and it works, KEEP IT LOCKED IN YOUR HEART!

Little moments as these will be moments to cherish forever.

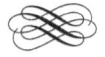

KATHERINE'S STORY:

When my mother is happy, she is very giddy and silly. She loves to sing and quote poetry. It amazes me that she can remember poems she learned in high school.

She also loves nature. She will always comment on trees and the beauty of flowers when I am driving her places. She and I are alike in that way. I treasure those conversations.

At my son's birthday party, she started to quote a few poems. Everyone enjoyed listening to her. A moment stood still for me, when my granddaughters ran to their room to get their Shel Silverstein books and began reading poetry to their grandmother.

MARIE'S STORY:

Fairy tales can come true, it can happen to you

If you're young at heart

For it's hard, you will find, to be narrow of mind

If you're young at heart

You can go to extremes with impossible schemes

You can laugh when your dreams fall apart at the seams

And life gets more exciting with each passing day

And love is either in your heart or on it's way

Don't you know that it's worth every treasure on earth

To be young at heart

For as rich as you are it's much better by far

To be young at heart

And if you should survive to 105

Look at all you'll derive out of being alive

Then here is the best part, you have a head start

If you are among the very young at heart

And if you should survive to 105

Look at all you'll derive out of being alive

Then here is the best part, you have a head start

If you are among the very young at heart

Songwriters

JOHNNY RICHARDS, CAROLYN LEIGH

At 94, my dad still has a beautiful voice. His favorite song to sing to my mom is "Young At Heart." I play a Perry Como version of the song every time I visit them. Both of them will sing, hold hands, and tap their feet. It's a memory I will always hold dear to my heart.

My dad stopped wearing his wedding band several years ago. His fingers were starting to bend due to the tendons in his hands shortening. When I was playing "Young at Heart," my mom turned to my dad and said, "You are not wearing your wedding band. If you don't, wear your's, I am not going to wear mine!" She gave a quick nod and looked at me for a reaction. I laughed. She continued with her conversation. "And, to let you know, Perry Como can leave his loafers on the floor next to my bed anytime he wants!" My dad looked at her and replied, "Is he still alive?!"

I have always tried to stay "young at heart". I find that when I visit I try to giggle and laugh as much as I can. I recall my dad saying to me he loves my laugh! To me, that is golden!

DANIEL'S STORY:

The bit of humor I find in my situation is that my mother is still in denial! She only thinks my father has the memory issues. The other day, she commented to me, "Your father is slipping. He is not as sharp as he used to be!"

On a beautiful sunny day, the three of us were sitting outside. My mother looked at my father and said he was getting old, since he was 89 years old.

My father replied, "Am I 89?"

I answered, "No. You are 87."

My mother chimed in, very insistently, "No. I'm 87, and he is 89!" She looked at him and said, "Don't you re-member the big party they had for me when I turned 87?"

My father, looking puzzled, "No, I don't remember."

I sat there smiling and watched them both. I thought to myself. "I, too, don't remember that party when she turned 87!" However, if she wants to think she is 87 and had a big party, then, so be it.

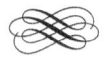

MICHAEL'S STORY:

A typical visit with my mother and father at their assisted living home:

"I'm hungry," he announces.

"Would you like some candy?" she offers.

"Yes. Do you have some?"

"No!"

"Helen?" No answer. "Can you hear me?"

"What?"

"Can you hear me?"

"No!"

"Where are your hearing aids?"

"What hearing aids? I don't wear hearing aids!"

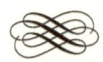

FELICIA'S STORY:

I have always had a healthy sense of humor. I use it with my mom all the time.

My mom wanted to lay down, so to make her more comfortable I suggested we take the necklaces off that she was wearing. As I was helping her to take off the necklaces, I started counting: "1,2, 3, 4, 5, 6, 7." She started laughing loudly. I asked her why she had worn so many necklaces. With that, she pulled another necklace out of her blouse!

"Oh, my goodness! What else do you have in there?" She started giggling like a child. She pulled out a pen, another necklace, and a folded piece of paper! We laughed and laughed. Not only did she have necklaces and other items down her blouse, she was also wearing two watches and three bracelets!

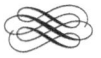

Chapter
Seven

IN MEMORY

Those we Love remain with us,
for Love itself lives on.
Cherished memories never fade,
because a loved one is gone.
Those we Love can never be,
more than a thought apart.
For as long as there is a memory,
they'll live on in our heart.

~Author unknown

GRACE'S STORY:

My grandma was born on August 11, 1926. She passed away April 8, 2013. She was one of those people who had to always keep busy. She was either working at her job, working on her house, or doing things for her family.

For many years, she and my grandpa owned a retail business in our hometown called The Lamp Shade House. People absolutely loved working with and for her at the store. Her nickname in town was "The Lamp Shade Lady." You could tell she loved participating in the daily operations of being a small business owner.

Growing up in the same town where she lived, my sister and I spent a lot of time with my grandma. She always had activities planned when we visited her. She would play, craft, and cook, right alongside of us. She was very active in her church, attending every Sunday and singing in the choir for many years. My grandma was a sharp lady. She was always happy and fulfilled in life.

I can remember the looks of frustration and fear when the first signs of her dementia appeared. She would forget my name or another family member's name. You could see her face drop. I can remember her desperate looks during conversations with my grandpa. It was clear they had both noticed her decline. However, she was in denial.

When my grandpa passed away, it was very difficult for my grandma living on her own. My parents had family discussions about moving my grandma from her home. However, we knew she would never move into an assisted living facility willingly. I think it was almost necessary to wait until something happened that gave her no choice.

The decision became apparent my grandmother could no longer drive. She bumped into a car in the grocery store parking lot and had difficulty exchanging information with the other driver and the police officer. My dad immediately took her keys and car from her. We all agreed it was the right decision.

It was heartbreaking to hear her stories of how she had started to walk places instead of calling for rides. She would walk across busy streets all over town to maintain her independence. Not long after the car was taken, she fell during one of her walking excursions. This incident led to her being put into a long term care facility. She never left.

I started to grieve for my grandma when she entered the facility. Every time I would leave after visiting, it would take me a while to forget the look of sadness, frustration, and fear in her face as I said goodbye. I could see in her eyes that she had so much to say to me, but no words would come. By that time, she wasn't able to comprehend yes/no questions. It was impossible to help fulfill the needs she very clearly had but could not express to me.

To watch the grandma I once knew as a lively and sharp lady decline, was very sad for me. I keep the memories close to my heart. I loved her very much.

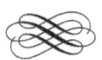

RHONDA'S STORY:

I was a caregiver for Mrs. Stevens, a woman who became family to me. I never realized she was an important part of my life until she passed. The grief I felt was something I had never experienced. I felt empty, lost and unimportant without her. She was a woman whose encouragement throughout my caregiving years with her I was happily received. I used to call her my cheerleader!

Mrs. Stevens was generally a quiet lady. She was more of an observer. However, I did not have to guess how she felt or what she thought. She would let it be known!

Not long after coming to care for her, I was folding her towels when I was informed it was NOT the Mrs. Stevens Way! While quietly watching, she suddenly told me, in her matter-of-fact manner, "I don't fold my towels that way!" She proceeded to show me how she wanted her towels folded. I still fold my own towels the Mrs. Stevens Way, with a smile on my face.

As her memory declined, she would forget names. We would work together for her to try and remember. She would maintain her positive spirit. I would often joke with Mrs. Stevens. She would sarcastically laugh, raise her eyebrow, and say, "Yeah, Riiiight!"

I would share with her my own stories. Many times, when I told her about how I exercised, her response would be "What would you want to do that for?" Mrs. Stevens did not like the thought of exercising! She preferred sitting and listening to classical music.

In her final years, Mrs. Stevens' dementia and eyesight worsened. Still, she never forgot who I was. When

I would arrive at her home, I would always say, "Hi, Mrs. Stevens! It's Rhonda!"

Her eyes would widen, and she would, ever so slightly lift her body to greet me, saying, "Oh, I'm so glad you're here. It's so nice to see you!" The way she said it was music to my ears.

I had other clients with dementia, but there was something about Mrs. Stevens. She is now gone. Losing someone I love was new and strange. It left me with a void in my life. I didn't know what to do. I believe, every person has a purpose in life. Mine is serving, and I think when we are not operating in that purpose, our life has no fulfillment.

I also believe that as human beings, we need validation. I have validation and love from my family. I have close and dear friends. I know they love me. But, for some reason, Mrs. Stevens made me feel special. I felt so validated by her. Her son at times would say that I was the daughter she never had. The only theory about our connection that I can offer, is that some people just bond together, and that bond can never be broken.

Mrs. Stevens loved coffee. It was her elixir! When she passed, I placed a bag of Starbucks "Tribute" coffee in her casket. I think the name is fitting for such an awesome woman. "Tribute" is a special edition that only comes out once a year. Each year, when it's displayed in stores, it is bittersweet for me. I drink a cup of the special blend in honor of the woman who was my cheerleader.

Grief, left me feeling lost. However, it has been replaced with the purpose for which I know God put me on this earth: to serve people who need assistance.

I still feel the loss and the void. I still cry and I still laugh. I am grateful for the memories I have of Mrs. Stevens. Not a day goes by without me thinking of her. I miss her dearly.

ELIZABETH'S STORY:

Sometimes our friends become our family.

My brother, John, was a pastor in Los Angeles. He became the head of the prison ministry for the cardinal.

Mother Teresa, the Catholic Sister and missionary, commonly known as a living saint, received a letter from a women in one of the prisons in which my brother held ministry. The woman asked Mother Teresa if she would visit the prison while she was in Los Angeles. John was asked to be Mother Teresa's escort. He escorted her to every venue. It was such an honor. One of the days, while flying in a helicopter over Los Angeles, John pointed out where our parents lived. She asked for a pencil and wrote a note to my parents on a brochure she had in her lap. She thanked them for giving their son to God, "He is a blessing to all of us." That brochure is framed and hangs proudly in my home since my brother passed.

I am very proud of my brother and all he did for others. My story will tell you how our friends became a lifeline of care.

Shortly after this most honorable time in my brother's life, he retired with three other priests to a home they purchased about an hour from any major city. Each summer, all the priests, except John, would leave the house for three weeks.

During those three weeks, every year, I would visit John. The summer of 2005, I noticed John was becoming forgetful. Two days before I was to leave, John asked me what was he going to do after I left.

I felt what we had set up for him, was sufficient, but

he was scared and finally admitted to me that he could not manage on his own any more. He had been trying to cover his decline while I was there with him. Now that I was leaving him, he had to make it known. He could no longer live on his own.

He was correct. I felt he needed long term care. There were no openings at the retirement center for priests. The bishop called a long term care facility in the town where my family was originally from. Thankfully, they had an opening for him.

I had a three-week commitment of mission work and couldn't change my dates. I didn't know what to do in regards of getting my brother moved into the nursing home. Our immediate family was just my brother and me.

This is where my friends became my family. A dear friend, Mary, who lived an hour away came to my aid. She packed John's belongings from the house and moved him to the nursing home.

I called my brother daily. After he was there for two weeks, I spoke to the staff nurse. She told me John was suddenly declining rapidly. He was starting to wander from section to section. The next step for John was in a locked ward for his safety.

Mary traveled with me to visit my brother when I came back from my mission trip. The new ward John lived in brought back his memories of the prison ministry. He would refer to the area he was living in as jail. During our visit, he kept insisting that we all go out to a restaurant. I couldn't possibly take him to a restaurant with the thought he was going back to "jail" afterwards!

After this visit, I made arrangements with the nursing staff that I would call daily. The nurse would give John the phone to talk with me.

Every two weeks, my cousin came from over an hour away to visit John. Each of those visits, she would bring his favorite Friendly's Ice Cream Sundae. She became part of what I call the "Fabulous Five"

Another one of my "Fabulous Five" was Mary Alice. Mary Alice knew John loved chocolate chip cookies with no nuts. Every visit, she brought her homemade cookies to John. Those cookies brought such a smile to John's face!

Friends Jean and Harold would visit. They were members of John's first church. Harold passed away not long after they began visiting John at the nursing home. However, Jean kept her commitment to John. She continued her visits with him. She knew John loved chocolates, and every two weeks, a visit from Jean was never without chocolate!

Another one of the "Fabulous Five" was Roberta, who worked with my brother. Roberta always had hard candies on her desk, which John loved. So, every visit, Roberta would make sure she brought some.

Over the two years my brother was in the nursing home, the "Fabulous Five" made sure he was not alone. They knew he was a Yankees fan and would always bring him clippings and memorabilia every visit. It would help spark a memory for him.

I tried to visit my brother every six weeks. For

financial reasons, that was all I was able to do. As I would say goodbye to my brother, he would say, "I know, six weeks!" John, eventually, began having no recollection of time.

Every visit, he knew who I was, until my last visit he did not know me. It was then, I knew he would not be here much longer.

There were many times of burden and struggles in living a far distance from my brother and tending to his needs. However, knowing I had the "Fabulous Five" to be my family support system gave me peace of mind.

My brother was an honorable man. He lived a full life. His unfortunate mental decline showed the enduring love in people's hearts. I have been truly blessed.

Allow yourself the acceptance of outside help.

Chapter

Eight

A dear friend of mine and I attend an annual conference sponsored by the Alzheimer's Association.

One of the most endearing and prevalent comments I heard from a wonderful speaker was this: **IT IS MORE IMPORTANT TO BE KIND THAN IT IS TO BE RIGHT.**

I think the following poem, written by an unknown author, brings light to her comment.

Do Not Ask Me to Remember

Do not ask me to remember,
Don't try to make me understand,
Let me rest and know you're with me,
Kiss my cheek and hold my hand.
I'm confused beyond your concept,
I am sad and sick and lost.
All I know is that I need you
To be with me at all cost.
Do not lose your patience with me,
Do not scold or curse or cry.
I can't help the way I'm acting,
Can't be different though I try.
Just remember that I need you,
That the best of me is gone,
Please don't fail to stand beside me,
Love me 'til my life is done.